Accountability

....

Deborah Glover

BSc, RGN

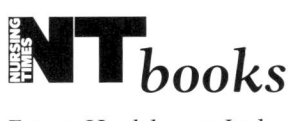

NT *books*

Emap Healthcare Ltd
Greater London House
Hampstead Road
London NW1 7EJ

Nursing Times Clinical Monographs are authoritative, concise, single subject publications designed to provide a critical review of material that will be of value to practising nurses, midwives and health visitors. Their authors, all experts in their field, are asked to be challenging and thought-provoking and to stimulate reflection on current practice. *Nursing Times* Clinical Monographs do not seek to be exhaustive reviews but up-to-date overviews; their critical and evaluative nature is designed to promote best practice through consideration of current evidence.

Topics for publication are decided by the editorial advisory board, with input from practitioners. Monographs are then commissioned as near as possible to the publication date to ensure that the information they contain is the latest available. All manuscripts are reviewed by a board member and a clinician working in the field covered.

At regular intervals, 12–15 new monographs will be published. They will cover subjects suggested by practitioners (see below) and any major new developments in the field of nursing care. Each publication will be on sale for a limited time, after which it will be withdrawn and, if necessary, replaced with an updated version.

Note: For referencing purposes NT Clinical Monographs should be treated as books

Suggestions for future titles are welcome and should be sent to Simon Seljeflot at NT Books, Emap Healthcare, Greater London House, London NW1 7EJ

All rights reserved. No part of this publication may be reproduced, stored in a retrieval system, or transmitted, in any form or by any means, electronic, mechanical, photocopying, recording or otherwise without the prior permission of the publisher.

Copyright © 1999 Emap Healthcare Ltd.

Study Hours

All NT Clinical Monographs have been given a Study Hours rating. This is an approximate guide to the amount of time it might take a nurse, midwife or health visitor with no specialist education on the subject to read and reflect on the article and consider the suggested key reading list. By doing this you can accrue Study Hours to help towards your PREP study activities. Make a note of any related study you undertake and keep a record in your personal professional profile. For your free Study Hours pack, call 01483 455040.

The Study Hours logo is a registered trade mark of Emap Healthcare Ltd.

Accountability

Deborah Glover, BSc, RGN

Nursing is a dynamic, complex and developing profession. As practitioners enhance their roles to incorporate aspects of patient care that were previously the domain of medical staff, their autonomy has necessarily increased. However, along with an increase in autonomy comes an increase in accountability. And, as accountable professionals, nurses must be able to explain and justify why they took the decisions they did during the course of their practice. All nurses need to know to whom they are accountable — the UKCC, the public, the patient and the employer. In some instances it will be all four. They also need to be aware of some of the basic issues in law that will guide their practice. Ignorance of the law is no excuse, nor is 'I was just following orders'. A thorough knowledge of accountability and its implications for practice will ensure that nurses will continue to develop their practice in response to patient and professional need in a safe and competent way

Background

The Nurse Registration Acts of 1919 were the result of some 30 years of vigorous campaigning by Mrs Bedford Fenwick and other members of the British Nurses' Association (comprising both matrons and doctors). They had already established a register of nurses who had undergone a year's training before 1889 and had the aim of state registration for nurses after three years' training (Baly, 1997).

This was in direct contrast to Florence Nightingale's wishes who felt that this would make nursing a 'profession rather than a calling' (Cook, 1913 — cited in Baly, 1997) and lower the standard.

However, the acts outlined and applied principles of nurse registration and regulation and gave rise to the General Nursing Councils. Thus the responsibility for and authority to ensure professional discipline and regulation has been vested in the statutory bodies for many years, along with a responsibility for the standards of training required by a nurse in order to register as a qualified practitioner.

However, it was only with the Nurses', Midwives' and Health Visitors' Act of 1979, which gave rise to the birth of the United Kingdom Central Council for Nursing, Midwifery and Health Visiting, that the level at which a registered nurse could perform was formalised through rule 18 of the act.

A mandatory requirement was placed on this new body to establish and improve standards of professional conduct and gave it the authority to do so, as set out in section 2(5) of the Nurses', Midwives' and Health Visitors' Act 1979: 'The powers of the council shall include that of providing, in such a manner as it sees fit, advice for nurses, midwives and health visitors on standards of professional conduct.'

With admirable foresight, the UKCC recognised that, as its main responsibility was to protect the public through standards for education, training and professional conduct, and that as nursing was becoming a developing, complex and dynamic profession, some guidance for practitioners would be beneficial. Additionally, it recognised that, as professional activity requires a degree of autonomy and independence in practice, personal accountability for these actions would be demanded. Accordingly, in 1984, the UKCC introduced the *Code of Professional Conduct* (which is now in its third edition) and other supporting documents over subsequent years.

The *Code of Professional Conduct* was the council's definitive advice on professional conduct to its practitioners (UKCC, 1992a). It was written to make explicit to practitioners the extent of their accountability and to assist them in the exercise of it.

The principle of accountability

Pennels (1997) defined accountability as being the 'requirement that each nurse is answerable and responsible for the outcome of his or her professional actions'.

She went on to say that the principle of accountability was an integral part of practice and that linked to this were three main points:
- It arises from the patient's expectation that, by virtue of a nurse's training and position, the nurse will be answerable to the patient while he or she is in their care;
- The principle that accountability arises from training and education explains why the notion is present in some jobs and not in others. Therefore, knowledge from training is essential in order to explain why an event took place;
- As accountability and authority are interdependent, a greater degree of accountability is expected of those with greater authority

To whom is the nurse accountable?

Although the *Code of Professional Conduct* outlines the professional accountability of the nurse as an individual and to the profession, nurses must be aware that there are others to whom they are accountable (see also section on nurse specialists).

Dimond (1995) stated that the nurse was accountable to the following:
- The **public** — through criminal law;
- The **employer** — through contract law — being answerable for breaches in the contract of employment or job description;
- The **patient** — through a duty of care and the common law of negligence and through civil law;
- The **profession** — through the *Code of Professional Conduct* and other relevant documents.

If a civil or criminal action is bought against a nurse they will be accountable simultaneously to the employer, the UKCC and the patient.

Indeed, the code alludes to these areas, as it states that each registered nurse, midwife and health visitor shall act, at all times, in such a manner as to safeguard and promote the interests of individual patients and clients, serve the interests of society, justify public trust and confidence and uphold and enhance the good standing and reputation of the profession

Accountability to the public
The NHS is mainly paid for through public taxation. Therefore, nurses are accountable to the public to provide a service for which they are employed and to use the available resources appropriately to provide that service.

However, conflicts may arise while trying to achieve this. For example, an employer may have decided that a certain wound dressing will be used in the organisation because it is the cheapest. Naturally, they will see this as being accountable for 'public' spending. However, nurses may know that the dressing is not necessarily the most effective. Therefore, they have to challenge its use, which risks conflict with their employer, but they have a professional responsibility to do this as well as accountability to the public to ensure they get the best value for their money.

Additionally, nurses are accountable to the public through criminal law. Criminal law is concerned with punishment for an offence rather than compensation. Therefore, it is unlikely that nurses will be sued by a patient under criminal law if their injuries are occasioned inadvertently or negligently (McHale et al, 1997). If however, nurses have deliberately or recklessly caused injury to them they may face charges under criminal law.

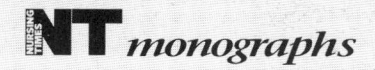

As with any member of the public, if nurses commit a crime they can be prosecuted for it — it is an offence against society. Therefore, if a nurse commits a criminal offence he or she is not 'serving the interests of society', as laid down in the *Code of Professional Conduct*. Accordingly, if a nurse is found guilty of a criminal offence there are systems in place that allow the police or the courts to report him or her to the Professional Conduct Committee. Similarly, if a nurse is brought before a PCC due to what could be a criminal offence (such as theft from a patient or unlawful wounding of a patient), then the UKCC can inform the appropriate authorities of this.

Accountability to the employer
Nurses are answerable to their employer through their contract of employment. The contract carries an implicit assumption that the employee will do what the employer wants by adhering to organisational policies, procedures and guidelines.

Nurses are also accountable for the proper and appropriate use of resources. For example, eating food designated for patients (even if they do not want it), using hospital stationery for personal use or undertaking an action not delegated to the nurse through the employer or one that is not accepted practice can lead to internal disciplinary action and/or reporting to the Professional Conduct Committee of the UKCC, especially if the actions have caused harm to a patient and he or she has taken an action for negligence.

Further issues arise in respect of accountability to employers. Copp (1988) stated that, in order for nurses to be accountable, they must have autonomy of action and authority to act within a defined nursing role. However, in most organisations nurses are not always able to exercise their autonomy and initiative. This is mainly due to the bureaucratic and hierarchical nature of the organisation and increasing fear of litigation.

At the end of the day, doctors are still legally responsible for the patient (NHS, 1992), so they will have to be involved in any decision as to what nurses can or cannot do within the course of their employment. Currently, the law supports this concept. The doctor diagnoses and prescribes, nurses carry out his orders (Hayward, 1999), unless they suspect negligence or criminal intent (such as euthanasia), when they would have to refuse to follow orders and make their concerns known.

Some of these restraints have been alleviated by the introduction and recognition of the *Scope of Professional Practice* (UKCC, 1992b). It has also served to further the autonomy and therefore the accountability of the nurse.

Scope of professional practice

Although historically and legally doctors have had overall responsibility for patients, they have 'allowed' nurses to undertake certain tasks through the process of delegation. These tasks were formalised under a Department of Health circular (Department of Health, 1997) that established the 'extended role' which allowed nurses to undertake certain tasks that were previously the domain of doctors. They had to be authorised by the employer, training had to be given, competence assessed and a certificate issued. This led, in many instances, to nurses collecting certificates for different tasks within their organisation. If they moved to another organisation, they usually had to undergo another training and assessment for the same task.

However, there was no on-going assessment of competence once the certificate was given and the range of tasks nurses could perform was restricted because hospital protocols prevented too many tasks being undertaken. Most of these restrictions were not in the patients' interests. For example, a nurse working in A&E could not plaster and nurses working in intensive care could not take arterial blood gases. This naturally led to delays in treatment, most notably in the administration of intravenous drugs.

Consequently, in 1992, the UKCC and government acknowledged the limitations of the extended role and introduced the *Scope of Professional Practice* (usually referred to as Scope). It recognised that nurses had the potential to develop their role to include aspects of care for which they did not necessarily hold certificates (Woodrow, 1996). Indeed, in response to Scope, the government withdrew the 1997 circular.

Woodrow (1996) argued that Scope refocused nursing into an autonomous profession able to make decisions for itself and take responsibility for its own actions. Thus, Scope further reinforced the concept of accountability.

Scope essentially requires that 'practice must be sensitive, relevant and responsive to patients needs . . . and have the capacity to adjust . . . to changing circumstances . . . the range and responsibilities which fall to individual nurses . . . should be related to their personal education, experience and skill' (UKCC, 1992b) and that these are achieved through the six principles outlined in the document.

Scope therefore has allowed nurses, midwives and health visitors to undertake tasks that were previously the remit of doctors, as long as the enhanced roles are in the best interests of the patient, not detrimental to fundamental nursing care and that the nurse is skilled and competent to do them.

Nurses also have to ensure that they maintain their competence (something not required previously) and acknowledge any limitations.

This means that employers have had to adapt to this concept in more ways than one. In order to take vicarious liability they have to approve any enhancement of the nurse's role, provide the relevant education and training and ratify the guidelines or protocols under which the nurse will work.

However, as Lunn (1994) argued, there is a dichotomy, as employers, through the employment contract, can still order nurses to undertake tasks not within their capabilities.

For example, an E-grade staff nurse may be asked to undertake the duties of an F grade in respect of patient assessment or administration of chemotherapy drugs, with the employers stating that they will back the nurse up if anything goes wrong. This, of course, would mean that the nurse is actually breaking her code of professional conduct if she accepts. It also begs the question: if the employer thinks the nurse is capable of doing the F grade job, why not train her up and give her the post?

Conscientious objection

This is an area where, again, nurses may come across conflict between their code and contract of employment. Clause 8 of the code requires nurses to 'report to an appropriate person . . . any conscientious objection which may be relevant to your particular practice' (UKCC, 1992a).

There are two specific areas to which conscientious objection can be legally raised — abortion, under the Abortion Act 1967, and technological procedures to achieve conception and pregnancy, under the Human Fertilisation and Embryo Act 1990.

Common sense would suggest that anyone who has a conscientious objection to these areas would choose not to work in them. However, because of shortages of beds many clinical areas are no longer 'dedicated', so nurses working in, for example, general surgery, may find patients who fall into these categories on their ward, or they may be deployed to work in these areas due to staff shortages. In these instances, nurses have to make their objection known as soon as possible. What should be remembered, however, is that the UKCC clearly states that in an emergency the nurse would be expected to provide care (UKCC, 1996).

Khan and Robson (1999) also suggested that there were some common law grounds where it may be in the

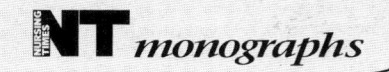

nurse's own interests not to participate, such as:
- Criminal acts — nurses can legally refuse to participate in a treatment or procedure they know is criminal in law — for example, the administration of a lethal injection for euthanasia purposes;
- Negligent acts — if asked to carry out a procedure nurses believe is likely to cause the patient harm — for example, giving the wrong dose of a drug;
- Withdrawing medical treatment — this is still a grey area and should be the subject of team and organisational discussion.

Vicarious liability

Generally, if nurses practise within the guidelines, protocols and terms of employment laid down by employers they will take vicarious liability if a nurse is negligent and a patient pursues a civil claim against him or her. This means that they will be held legally responsible for the nurse's actions, provided they were undertaken during the course of employment. Vicarious liability is said to derive from the 1711 Servants Charter Act, the principle being: 'Let the master answer'.

An example of an organisation's policy statement on vicarious liability is the following: "Nurses are under a duty to exercise reasonable care when carrying out their employment. The employing authority will be vicariously liable for and will provide indemnity to nurses in respect of any legal proceedings based upon a breach of their duty of care. This organisation therefore will continue to accept vicarious liability for any nurse who acts in good faith in the course of their employment. Naturally, any apparent failure to exercise reasonable care and skill may result in the invoking of investigation and/or disciplinary procedures internally and by the relevant professional and legal bodies.'

Accountability to the patient
This is arguably the most important area of a nurse's accountability. It is central to the function of the UKCC, as it exists to protect the public and does so by providing standards of education, training and professional conduct for its registrants.

As autonomous practitioners, nurses are answerable and responsible for the outcome of their professional action. They have a legal and professional duty to ensure that they care for their patients and that the care was given to a certain standard.

The nurse's duty of care

Traditionally, the legal test of a duty of care is based on the 'neighbour principle' and arose out of a case in which a young woman sued a soft drinks manufacturer after finding a partially decomposed snail in a bottle of ginger beer she had begun to drink (Donoghue v Stevenson, 1932).

The neighbour principle is based on a statement made by Lord Aitkin during the case: 'You must take reasonable care to avoid acts or omissions which you can reasonably foresee would be likely to injure your neighbour.'

In other words, people have a duty of care to another if they can see that their actions are reasonably likely to cause harm to another person. Therefore, nurses have a duty of care to their patients by virtue of the nurse/patient relationship that they and the patient enter into.

However, a duty of care is not absolute and will vary according to situation. A duty of care is discharged when a nurse does what is reasonable in a particular set of circumstances, where 'reasonableness' is the standard set by law.

If a duty of care is breached in some way, either through act or omission, a civil action for negligence may be brought by the patient.

Hepple and Matthews (1991) stated that the tort of negligence has been subject to a variety of classifications, but the fundamental elements are said to be that a duty of care is owed, a breach in that duty of care occurred and the breach caused reasonably foreseeable harm.

The legal duty of care, however, does not apply at all times and in all places. For the duty to exist there needs to be a pre-existing relationship. It applies once the patient has accepted treatment or presented himself for potential treatment, such as coming into hospital, using the services of the GP, practice nurse or community nurse.

Therefore, if a nurse were walking to the shops and saw someone collapsed in the street, he or she would not be legally required to stop and give assistance, as there is no pre-existing relationship. However, once the nurse gives assistance, it will have to be of the standard outlined below. Nurses do, however, have a professional duty as laid down by the UKCC in the code to 'serve the interests of society, justify public trust and confidence and uphold the good standing and reputation of the professions'.

The standard of care

The court determines what would have been a reasonable action in a particular set of circumstances through the application of the Bolam test, described as follows: 'The test is the standard of the ordinary skilled man exercising and professing to have that special skill. A man need not possess the highest expert skill at the risk of being found negligent . . . it is sufficient if he exercises the ordinary skill of an ordinary competent man exercising that particular art' (Bolam v Friern Barnet Hospital Management Committee, 1957).

For example, a surgeon would need to exercise the ordinary special skill of a surgeon and a physician the ordinary special skill of a physician.

The Bolam test arose out of case law relating specifically to doctors, but its principles apply to all health care professionals, including nurses. Pennels (1998) stated that the principle of competence went hand in hand with accountability because:
● There is an expectation that on completion of basic training the knowledge gained should enable the nurse to function safely;
● The patient should be able to reasonably rely on the practitioner's position and registration in assuming that he or she is competent to care for him or her.

This competence and the Bolam test may, of course, be revised in the light of developments in nursing roles that have arisen as a consequence of the *Scope of Professional Practice* (UKCC, 1992b).

This principle applies to all qualified nurses, regardless of grade or level of experience. In law, being inexperienced is no defence to an action being brought, and learners or trainees are judged at the same standard as a more experienced colleague.

This was demonstrated in Nettleship v Weston (1971), where it was held that a learner driver must meet the standard of care of a qualified driver, even *vis-à-vis* the standard of his instructor.

If, however, advice was sought from a more senior or experienced person, then accountability has been discharged and the more senior practitioner is accountable.

The test case for this principle was that of Wilsher v Essex Area Health Authority (1986). A senior house officer inserted an umbilical arterial catheter into a baby's vein instead of an artery, thus giving false oxygen saturation readings. He asked his registrar to check the catheter position. The registrar replaced it, but again into a vein. The baby received too much oxygen and as a result contracted retrolental fibroplasia. The judge stated that the SHO was not negligent, as he was entitled to have his worked checked by a senior.

However, and perhaps more importantly, it was ruled that doctors and nurses have a duty of care related to the post they hold and the task performed. This has implications for specialists practitioners, as will be discussed later.

It must also be recognised that employers have a responsibility to ensure that the person in post is competent, and they may be directly liable if staff are placed in situations that they were not competent to be in. Nevertheless, this does not detract from a nurse's professional accountability to acknowledge the limitations of her competence (Furlong and Glover, 1998a).

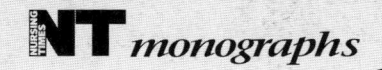

In practice, issues can arise in which the nurse must be aware of her accountability. These include delegation, consent and confidentiality.

Delegation

Nurses are accountable for the decision to delegate and for ensuring that the task delegated has been undertaken. As mentioned before, doctors, under the *Terms of Service for Doctors* (NHS, 1992), are responsible for the patient. They can, however, delegate to a person 'whom they have authorised and who they are satisfied is competent to carry out such treatment'. Therefore, nurses are obliged morally, if not legally, to delegate to a competent person (Glover, 1999).

In the course of practice, nurses are likely to delegate to a number of people.

Students
Students are protected form full accountability until they have qualified. However, they are still responsible for their actions. Accountability for a delegated activity still rests with the registered nurse who delegated. Therefore, it is essential that qualified nurses are aware of the limitations of students and what they can and cannot do. This, of course, is not so easy with student on the Project 2000 syllabus, as their experience and skills are not as clear-cut for each ward placement as they used to be under the 'apprenticeship' training.

Heath care support workers
Again, with HCSWs competencies can vary according to the level of the National Vocational Qualification they have undertaken and where they have undertaken it. The delegating nurse must satisfy him or herself of the level of skill of the HCSW before delegating tasks.

Team members
In law, there is no concept of team liability. All (qualified) individuals within a team are personally and professionally accountable. Again, as team leaders nurses must satisfy themselves of the others' competence.

Relatives
Increasingly, patients are being discharged home with complex needs. In many instances, it falls to relatives to care for both the patient and the accompanying equipment and treatment regimes such as nasogastric feeding, intravenous drug administration or care of central lines. Nurses must satisfy themselves that that relatives are able to undertake this care and that they are happy to do so.

With regard to personal practice, the code of professional practice, clause 4, states that nurses must 'decline any duties [they] feel unable to perform in a safe and skilled manner'.

Once nurses have done this, they have discharged their accountability requirements.

Consent

Nurses are accountable for ensuring that the patient has given consent for any treatment they are giving. Much of the nursing care undertaken is done with implied consent — for example, the patient will roll up his sleeve if a nurse approaches with a sphygmomanometer or open his mouth to have his temperature taken.

It is, however, worthwhile remembering that under civil and criminal law, treating without consent can lead to charges of assault — where the patients is 'in fear' of physical contact without his or her consent — or battery — where the patient is actually touched or treated without permission (Pennels, 1998).

Clauses 1, 2 and 7 of the code of professional conduct relate to nurses' accountability in respect of consent. Consent, even implied consent, should be obtained only after the nurse has given the patient adequate information in order for him or her to make a meaningful decision (UKCC, 1996). If the nurse is performing the procedure, he or she should be the one to obtain the consent, except in an urgent situation when someone else can obtain it for them. Nurses must be satisfied that the person was competent to give the patient the information required to gain the consent.

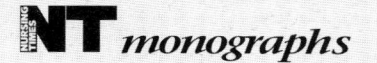

The information nurses give to patients before obtaining consent should do the following:
- Conform with that which a responsible body of similar professionals in the same specialty would give the patient;
- Inform the patient about the nature of the procedure;
- Inform the patient of the 'material risks' of the procedure — that is, those risks to which a reasonable patient would attach some significance;
- Be dictated by circumstance;
- Be given without undue influence or duress.

Competent adults can refuse consent. However, if they are suspected to be mentally unfit to give it, this refusal can be overruled by the court. For example, in Re T (1992), where a pregnant Jehovah's witness refused a blood transfusion after going into premature labour and thus needing a Caesarean section, her refusal was overturned by the court in order to protect the baby and the mother.

No person can given consent for another (adult) person, and relatives cannot legally give consent for another person, except in cases of emergency or mental incompetence. However, this will require a court order.

Similarly, nurses cannot withhold information from patients unless the doctor deems it to be detrimental to their well-being. Therefore, relatives cannot ask a nurse 'not to tell Mum she has cancer'.

In the case of children, the UKCC (1996) advises that, as consent of patients under 16 is complex, nurses should follow local protocols and legislation that affects their treatment. Similarly, the same should apply to those who are mentally incapacitated and those sectioned under the Mental Health Acts.

Confidentiality

Clause 10 of the code deals with this issue by requiring all nurses to 'protect all confidential information concerning patients . . . obtained in the course of professional practice and make disclosures only with consent where required by the order of a court or where you can justify disclosure in the wider public interest' (UKCC, 1992a).

There are, however, exceptions to the duty of confidentiality, which are by consent, by law, in the public interest or required by the police.

Consent
This may be implied or expressed. Implied usually refers to the fact that information regarding patients can be passed between professionals caring for them, but patients should be aware that this will happen. This sharing of information should happen only on a 'need to know' basis. Therefore, non-health care professionals — for instance, visiting clergy — have no right to read patients' notes without their consent.

Express consent may be obtained in response to circumstances, such as telling a relative or friend or the media about the patient's condition.

Law
Nurses have to disclose or withhold information according to certain statutes or specific court orders. These are:
- **Statutory duty to disclose information:**
Abortion Act 1992;
Misuse of Drugs Act 1971;
Public Health Act 1984;
Prevention of Terrorism Act 1988;
Road Traffic Act 1972.
- **Statutory duty to withhold information:**
NHS Venereal Diseases Act 1974;
Human Fertilisation and Embryo Act 1990.
- **Court Orders:**
Usually in a civil claim for negligence. The court can order either or both parties to disclose any relevant information or documentation.

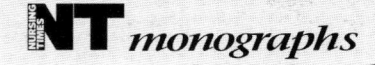

Public interest

The UKCC (1996) defines public interest to be 'the interests of an individual, or group of individuals, or of a society as a whole and would . . . cover matters such as serious crime, child abuse, drug-trafficking or other activities which could place others at serious risk'.

Whatever the situation a nurse may be in, he or she must be able to justify giving or withholding information and, as always, it must be documented.

The police

The police can gain access to information under procedures laid down in Schedule 1 of the Police and Criminal Evidence Act 1984.

Accountability to the profession

As mentioned earlier, the code requires that a registered nurse must 'act in such a manner as to justify public trust and confidence . . . and uphold and enhance the good standing and reputation of the profession' (UKCC, 1992a).

This, in effect, means that nurses have to act in a professional way whether currently engaged in practice or not and whether on or off duty. Therefore, any registered nurse who, for example, decides to take part in a programme about his or her antics on holiday or is drunk and disorderly while in uniform could be seen to be breaking the code.

Clauses 3, 6, 13 and 14 also relate to accountability to the profession. Clause 3 states that nurses must 'maintain and improve [their] professional knowledge and competence' (UKCC, 1992a).

Here, nurses are accountable for keeping themselves up to date in order to ensure that they are competent practitioners and because they will be passing knowledge on to their peers and subordinates.

Additionally, if nurses do not keep up to date they will be accountable if a case of negligence were brought against them. In the case of Hepworth v Kerr (1995) it was found that the defendant had failed to keep up to date with a particular procedure and so he was found negligent. However, it is acknowledged that one cannot possibly read every text as soon as it is published. The guiding principle must be that nurses must be up to date with regard to their area of practice and be aware of developments in other areas that may affect their practice.

Clause 6 states that they must 'work in a collaborative manner with health care professionals . . . and respect their particular contribution' (UKCC, 1992a). This is self-explanatory. Nurses cannot expect to know everything and therefore are reliant on others for information.

Clause 13 states 'report to an appropriate person . . . where it appears that the health and safety of colleagues is at risk . . . as circumstances may compromise . . . care' (UKCC, 1992a).

Again, this is self-explanatory. Although it may superficially appear that nurses are asked to inform on a friend or colleague, in reality they are helping them and, therefore, indirectly the patient, and discharging their accountability requirements. By caring for a fellow professional, nurses are protecting them from possible further harm or, indeed, from legal or professional redress.

Clause 14 states that nurses must 'assist professional colleagues . . . to develop their professional competence' (UKCC, 1992a).

All nurses have a responsibility to help colleagues through explicit teaching, clinical supervision or moral support.

Clinical supervision

This helps nurses develop skills and knowledge through reflection, support and guidance. However, the supervisor and the supervisee both have accountability and responsibilities within this process.

Supervisors have a professional and contractual duty to report any information given within the supervision session that may constitute a danger to patients (Dimond, 1998).

Although the principle of supervision is that the supervisor helps the supervisee explore issues and alternatives, supervisors must also be aware of the advice they give. It must not be negligent.

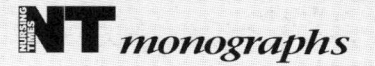

If the supervisee is seen to be a danger to the patient and the supervisor does not take any action, he or she will be held accountable if the patient is harmed. If the supervisee feels that the supervisor is giving poor or negligent advice, he or she is accountable for letting someone in authority know. This is in order to protect other colleagues the person may be supervising and, indirectly, to protect the patient.

Dimond (1998) summed up the accountability issues in supervision as follows:
● During supervision, any information disclosing danger to a patient must be followed up;
● Principles of law regarding liability should be taken into account where clinical supervision is practised;
● The supervisee has the same duties in terms of accountability as the supervisor;
● Confidential information may be passed on during clinical supervision, and this should be made clear to the patient;
● Clinical supervision records may have to be produced under subpoena;

Specialist practitioners

Over recent years the nursing profession has seen a growth in what can be termed 'specialist practitioners'. These include clinical nurse specialists, night practitioners, nurse practitioners and so on. As has already been mentioned, the accountability of these practitioners may be greater than that of the 'ordinary' practitioner.

Pennels (1998) argued that 'in the eyes of the law, nurses who profess to be trained in, to have experience of and to practice a specialty are regarded differently from nurses who do not claim such a specialist position'. In addition, the UKCC, patients and the law will expect much more.

Indeed, this was held in the case of Wilsher v Essex Area Health Authority (1988), where it was judged that the standard of care one would be expected to achieve is that of the post held and not the person holding the job. So if a nurse is in a post or undertaking duties previously held by a doctor — for example, undertaking endoscopies or patient physical assessment — the standard of care required would be that of a doctor and not a nurse.

The principle here is that specialists are expected to deliver a higher standard of care which reflects their additional training and experience and the fact that they occupy a specialist post. They must also have all the skills required for the job, and current accepted practice in the specialism must guide practice.

However, a note of caution must be added. It is documented that many specialist nurses have differing levels of education and training (Furlong and Glover, 1998b; Kaufman, 1996; Doyal, 1998; Dowling et al, 1996). Therefore, they may not always be cognisant of the above.

Pennels (1998) also suggested that specialists are also accountable to or for the following:
● The team — although there is no concept of team liability, individuals are accountable and the specialist nurse must be aware of the skill mix and competence of others;
● Delegation — specialists are often leaders, therefore they delegate. They must do this appropriately and not allow misuse of their position by undertaking work delegated to them by other health professionals which is outside their remit;
● Use of information — information given should conform to that which a responsible body of similar professionals in the same specialty would tell the patient;
● Documentation — specialists may wish to devise documentation specific to their specialty in which important details can be recorded.

A note of caution: specialists working independently are more accountable for their practice. Young (1994) cited the case of Sutton v Population Services 1981, where a nurse employed in a family planning clinic failed to notice, or act on evidence of, a lump in a patient's breast and was held to be negligent.

In terms of consent, patients may not be aware to whom they are giving consent and consequently who they understand will be undertaking the procedure.

Furlong and Glover (1998c) illustrated this as follows: 'When the Spanish *conquistadors* arrived in Mexico and dismounted from their horses, the indigenous population thought that they were seeing creatures who could split in two at will. Likewise, there are some new nursing roles that are so far removed from their origins that there may be few clues (such as uniform, title or actions) to help patients to identify incumbents as nurses.

'Differing perceptions of who health care professionals in new roles are may have implications in terms of the consent given by the patient. In law, any unauthorised touching of a patient when, for example, a patient assumes that the nurse is a doctor, is technically a battery and a civil claim can be made, even if there is no evidence of damage to the plaintiff. Do patients realise that they are consenting to an examination performed by a nurse, not by a doctor? If they had, would they have consented? sented?'

Conclusion

Accountability is like pregnancy — you cannot be slightly pregnant and you cannot be slightly accountable. The concept of accountability in nursing has been in place for many years. However, it is only since the advent of the UKCC and with self-regulation that it has come to the fore in most nurses' minds.

That said, there are still many nurses who are unaware of their accountability or confused by the concept as it applies to them. It is imperative, therefore, that the *Code of Professional Practice* and other UKCC documents are studied and applied to practice.

Unfortunately, the principles contained in the code are not always clear cut, and application may be difficult. However, nurses must be aware of all aspects of their accountability and to whom they are accountable and act accordingly.

Ultimately, no matter how many people tell you that they will back you if you 'do X, just this once', once you have done it and it goes wrong you are the accountable one and the others will have disappeared into the ether. It is better to not have a job but still be on the register than have no job and no career. **NT**

References

Baly, M. (1997) *Florence Nightingale and the Nursing Legacy*. London: Whurr Publishers.

Bolam v Friern Barnet Hospital Management Committee (1957) ALL ER 118.

Copp, G. (1988) Professional accountability; the conflict. *Nursing Times*; 84: 43, 42–44.

Cresswell, J. (1998) Accountability in prescribing. *Nurse Prescriber/Community Nurse*; 3: 41–42.

Department of Health (1971) *Health Circular. HC 77 (22)*. London: HMSO

Dimond, B. (1995) *Legal Aspects of Nursing*. London: Prentice Hall.

Dimond, B. (1998) Legal aspects of clinical supervision 2: professional accountability. *British Journal of Nursing*; 7: 8, 487–489.

Donoghue v Stevenson (1932) AC 562.

Doyal, L. (1998) Crossing professional boundaries. *Nursing Management*; 5: 4, 8–10.

Dowling, S., Martin, R., Skidmore, P., Doyal, L. (1996) Nurses taking on junior doctors' work: a confusion of accountability. *British Medical Journal*; 312: 7040, 44–47.

Furlong, S., Glover, D. (1998a) Legal accountability in changing practice. *Nursing Times*; 94: 39, 61–62.

Furlong, S., Glover, D. (1998b) Confusion surrounds piecemeal changes in nurses' roles. *Nursing Times*; 94: 37, 54–55.

Furlong, S., Glover, D. (1998c) Consent, equity and ethics in new nursing. *Nursing Times*; 94: 33, 52–53.

Glover, D. (1999) To do or not to do. In: Heywood-Jones, I. (ed) *The UKCC Code of Conduct: A Critical Guide*. London: NT Books

Hayward, M. (1999) Tug of war. *Nursing Times*; 95: 29, 28–29.

Hepple, B.A., Matthews, M.H. (1991) *Tort Cases and Materials*. London: Butterworth.

Hepworth v Kerr (1995) 6 Med LTR 139.

Kaufman, G. (1996) Nurse practitioners in general practice. *Nursing Standard*; 11: 8,

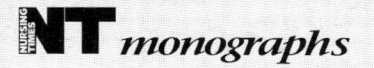

44–47.

Khan, M., Robson, M. (1999) A Matter of Conscience: In: Heywood-Jones, I. (ed) *The UKCC Code of Conduct: A Critical Guide.* London: NT Books.

Lunn, J. (1994) The *Scope of Professional Practice* from a legal perspective. *British Journal of Nursing*; 4: 16, 948–952.

McHale, J., Fox, M., Murphy, J. (1997) *Health Care Law Texts: Cases and Materials.* London: Sweet and Maxwell.

Nettleship v Weston (1971) 3 ALL ER 581.

NHS (General Medical Services) *Regulations SI (1992) 1992/636 Schedule 2: Terms of Service for Doctors (regulations 3 [2]).* London: Department of Health.

Nurses', Midwives' and Health Visitors' Act 1979. London: HMSO.

Pennels, C. (1997) Nursing and the law: clinical responsibility. *Professional Nurse*; 13: 3, 162–164.

Pennels, C. (1998) *Nursing and the Law.* London: Professional Nurse/EMAP Healthcare.

Re T [1992] Court of Appeal; 3 Med LR 306; 4 ALL ER 649.

UKCC (1992a) *Code of Professional Conduct.* London: UKCC.

UKCC (1992b) *The Scope of Professional Practice.* London: UKCC.

UKCC (1996) *Guidelines for Professional Practice.* London: UKCC

Wilsher v Essex Area Health Authority (1986) 3ALL E 801 [1987] I QB 730 [1987] 2 WLR 425.

Woodrow, P. (1996) Professional practice; the impact of the UKCC practice principles. *Nursing Standard*; 10: 49, 39–41.

Young, AP. (1994) *Law and Professional Conduct in Nursing.* London: Scutari Press.

Further reading

Khan, M., Robson, M. (1997) *Medical Negligence.* London: Cavendish Publishing.

Heywood-Jones, I. (1999) (ed) *The UKCC Code of Conduct: A Critical Guide.* London: NT Books.

Montgomery, J. (1997) *Healthcare Law.* Oxford: Oxford University Press.

Pennels, C. (1998) *Nursing and the Law.* London: Professional Nurse/EMAP Healthcare.

Pyne, R.H. (1981) *Professional Discipline in Nursing, Midwifery and Health Visiting.* Oxford: Blackwell Scientific.

Tingle, J., Cribb, A. (Eds) (1990) *Nursing Law and Ethics.* Oxford: Blackwell Science.

Young, A.P. (1993) *Legal Problems in Practice.* London: Chapman Hall.